FREE MEDICINE

6 SPS HEALTHY HABITS

Live Long Healthy Like A Turtle

6 Super Powerful Simple Secret Habits
for Health and Wellness

GRACE PRABHA

Disclaimer

The strategies presented in this book are for informational and educational purposes only; they are not substitute for professional counseling. Seek guidance from a qualified professionals for personalized support.

If you choose to use any information from this book for personal use, which is your constitutional right, the author assumes no responsibility for your actions.

Contents

I Introduction

"He who has health, has hope; and he
who has hope, has everything."
— Ancient Sanskrit Proverb

In the age of AI and bots, the mantra **"Health is Wealth"** resonates more than ever. We're surrounded by an array of options—from dieting and exercise to naturopathy, traditional yoga, meditation, and modern therapy programs—all aimed at enhancing our physical and mental well-being. I'm sure many of us have dabbled in a few.

Surprisingly, there are over 240 medical therapies globally, armed with advanced sciences. Yet, there are still individuals seeking that elusive cure and care. Can you believe it? It begs the question: Is there something missing in the pursuit of well-being, health, and happiness, beyond external treatments?

Allow me to share a tale my grandma used to spin when I was little—a story that holds timeless wisdom for all of us. Let's rewind and bask in its goodness together.

In a distant realm, Emperor Venus reigned in opulence, overseeing a populace basking in happiness and good health.

The monarch had two sons, and while one was a charming lad with a penchant for questioning everything, he found the strict regimen of good habits imposed upon him somewhat irksome. Frustrated, he expressed his bewilderment to his father, questioning the necessity of such disciplined practices.

Sensitive to his son's predicament, the king took a subtle approach. The next day, he enlisted the wisdom of a courtier to enlighten the prince on the significance of cultivating good habits.

The wise man gifted the prince a few exotic plants, emphasizing that their well-being was crucial for the prosperity of the kingdom. The prince, initially intrigued, diligently cared for the plants, witnessing their growth with pride.

However, life's distractions led him to neglect the plants during a countrywide tour. Upon his return, he found the once-thriving plants now withered and tired. The wise man seized this moment to impart a valuable lesson.

"Dear prince," he mused, "our good habits are akin to these fortune plants. The effort we invest in nurturing them determines the benefits they yield. Just as these plants require consistent care, so do our habits."

The prince, enlightened and grateful, recognized the importance of regular practice in cultivating both plants and good habits.

This tale underscores the myriad habits ingrained in us throughout life, shaped by customs, rituals, and family values. They serve as the essential life hacks from the moment we set foot on this Earth until we depart, even lingering beyond the departure of our souls, illuminating our humble abode with a divine glow.

From the rituals of infant bathing, head shaving, ear piercing, to naming ceremonies – every daily, seasonal, and annual routine, including festivals, holds inherent value for our well-being.

Back in my childhood, I was roused at the crisp hour of 5 am every morning, whether or not I had any pressing tasks. I often pondered the wisdom of waking up so early to gaze at the blue sky. As an energetically curious child, I'd plead with my grandma, saying, "Give me some task; I can take it to the sky and handle it, you'll see." Her response was always, "Just wait and watch. Your turn to take on responsibilities will come soon."

She was spot-on. Today, at the ripe age of over 95, she sits in the courtyard, gazing at the sky, quipping, "Your turn to work has arrived, and I'm content to watch." I realize that her enduring health and mental fortitude are a testament to the wisdom embedded in her daily practices.

As a practitioner in alternative medicine, I easily connect the dots, recognizing the paramount importance of cultivating healthy habits for robust well-being.

What seemed like pointless traditions back in the day are turning out to be hidden gems of health wisdom in today's age. Take, for example, the taboo against crossing your legs. Turns out, sitting in that position for extended periods can obstruct blood flow, disrupt the natural flow of Saram (Swara) in the body, and mess with the positioning of the femur bone. Particularly for women post-delivery, it's not recommended as it might introduce air into the body through the birth canal.

Another frowned-upon practice was leg shaking while sitting. Now I get it – a lot of nerve-related issues, from varicose veins to sciatica, can be traced back to the restless leg syndrome. Through seemingly simple customs, our ancestors inadvertently handed down a guidebook for maintaining good health.

The keys to a healthy life, as per the study, encompass various factors:

- Cultivating healthy habits
- Nurturing the well-being of body, mind, and soul
- Engaging in exercises, yoga, or comprehensive joint movements and muscle stretches

- Fostering a joyous mindset
- Exploring natural remedies
- Connecting with nature

In the current era, we're increasingly attuned to the significance of exercises and yoga for our overall well-being. However, the importance of healthy habits often takes a back seat, even though they serve as the bedrock. Think of it as building a strong foundation for a structure – when the base is robust, all the embellishments fall into place seamlessly.

This book is a spotlight on the top six healthy habits crucial for ensuring our long-term health and happiness. Get ready to embrace a lifestyle that not only enhances your well-being but also sets the stage for a flourishing future.

My Journey

My journey into the world of yoga commenced with Simple Kundalini Yoga (SKY), long before wrapping up my undergraduate studies. Initially, all was well – a handful of daily practices kept me both healthy and mindful. However, life took a turn after marriage, introducing relocation, new projects at work, and the formidable challenge of carving out "me time." The hustle and bustle of life swept away my commitment to health practices, and for a while, the busy routine seemed sustainable, clocking in at 4 am and out to bed at 12 am.

Then, reality hit. A few miles into a walk, back pain emerged, triggering a reminder of my abandoned health routine. This prompted my return to a yoga class. Yet, the wake-up call was more dramatic; attempting to rise while playing with my kids, I heard the creak of my backbones and found myself unconscious. In that moment, I coached myself: "Breathe! All is going to be good. Keep breathing." A paralysis attack left me bedridden for a month due to lumbar degeneration.

This challenging period became a profound "Health is Wealth" moment, an enlightenment born out of situation. Through unwavering effort, support from healthy habits, and various treatments, including yoga, acupuncture, dorn, and homeopathy, I slowly recovered. The experience inspired me to delve into a broader understanding of health and wellness, prompting me to embark on an alternative medicine and therapy courses.

As life returned to normalcy, so did responsibilities and duties. Managing time for a one-hour exercise routine proved challenging, echoing sentiments from associates. Thus began my quest for efficient time management and the birth of a unique health program. Drawing on my knowledge of various techniques, I crafted a fitness regimen that takes less than ten minutes, offering a holistic approach to health and mindfulness.

Now, I not only respect Mother Nature but also advocate for a sustainable lifestyle. Through my journey, I've learned, recovered, and grown – embracing the philosophy that health truly is wealth.

I have lined up all these six super powerful exercises in my book "Free Medicine: 6 Super Powerful Simple Health Yoga Techniques". Dive into it, master these techniques, and empower your body and mind for enduring health.

As these exercises keep our joints and muscles agile so that they don't get rusted, our inner cleanliness is needed to keep our organs, reservoirs and related canals free from sedimentations. This cleansing is needed every day, or many times a day, to be precise, as often as possible.

Note: *In the realm of therapy, we embrace a holistic view of the body—no isolating issues based on diseases. The names and descriptions of ailments often instill more fear than the actual* *impact. That's why, in this book, I focus solely on fostering a positive, healthy outlook through good habits rather than framing them as remedies for specific diseases. It's all about cultivating a wellness mindset!.*

This book shines a light on powerful yet simple healthy habits, often overlooked for their incredible benefits. It serves as your roadmap to seamlessly integrate these habits into your daily routine, paving the way for a healthier life.

Think of this book as your go-to guide for practical advice rather than a dry collection of scientific data sheets. There's a plethora of research and facts available elsewhere, complete with data-driven graphs and references. This book's goal is to distill the essential habits that can universally contribute to better health.

I earnestly urge my readers to embrace the methods presented here, experience the benefits firsthand, and recognize their significance.

Loaded with actionable assignments, use this book as your daily companion on the journey to better health—get ready to take on these assignments and make them a regular part of your routine.

II Lets Meet Habits

> "We are what we repeatedly do. Excellence,
> then, is not an act, but a habit."
>
> **— Will Durant**

A habit is like a well-worn path—it's a routine process etched into the grooves of our subconscious mind. Over time, our minds seamlessly adopt it, functioning automatically without conscious effort.

Embarking on something new often involves repetition until it effortlessly becomes second nature. We engage in the process repeatedly, and before we know it, it seamlessly integrates into our daily rhythm—much like our breath or heartbeat. It transforms into a habit.

When it comes to habits, two crucial aspects stand out:

1. **Cultivating the Right Habits**
2. **Correcting Old Habits to the Right Ones**

Establishing the right habits requires consistent practice, a conscious effort to ingrain them into our routine. Surprisingly, building new habits is not only easy but even easier than redirecting entrenched old habits. So, let's navigate the journey of cultivating and refining our habits with intention and commitment.

Cultivating the Right Habits

Embarking on the journey of building a habit for the first time on this planet? Here's the game plan:

* **Define your Objective** : Set an achievable goal
* **Find the process** : Chart out the process to achieve your goal

* **Repeat** : Repeat the process regularly

1. Set an achievable goal:

Specify a target that packs a punch in the benefits department once it becomes a habit.

Consider this - setting a goal like having your mom wake you up at 5 am daily might sound appealing, but it's not exactly feasible. Dependence on someone else could easily break this habit or worse, strain your relationship. Opt for a goal like consistently waking up at 5 am. It's within your control, no matter the circumstances.

Take into account all the factors influencing your goal. If your work routine has you burning the midnight oil until 12 am, aiming to rise at 5 am might not be realistic. It's not just about waking up early; it's about ensuring you get a healthy amount of sleep. Adjust your goal accordingly – perhaps aim to hit the hay by 10 pm and rise at 5 am after a rejuvenating night's sleep. This might open doors to a new job or even prompt flexibility in your current one.

And here's a **golden rule** – make it a goal to always opt for the healthier choice in all aspects of life. Prioritizing your health in every decision sets the stage for the mind that values well-being just as much as any other life choice. So, buckle up for the journey of crafting habits that not only stick but elevate your overall lifestyle.

2. Chart out the process to achieve your goal:

Plotting the course to your goal is like drawing up a treasure map – you've got to have a clear path, right?

Enter the process, the roadmap to your aspirations. Break it down into bite-sized milestones for that sweet taste of accomplishment. Celebrate each milestone, savoring the success stories that fuel your motivation.

Make this journey a blast—infuse it with fun, enjoyment, and sprinkle in rewards. After all, conquering your goals should feel like an epic adventure!

3. Repeat the process regularly:

Keep at it consistently—genuinely, a lot of us hit a snag here.

Let me lay it out straight. If you're not staying consistent, it suggests your goal might not be as beneficial as you think. Embrace flexibility, but do so with responsibility. Seek out social support; whether it's a group, a friend, or a family member, having someone in your corner is key to sticking with your routine.

It boils down to revisiting the four laws of behavior change: make it clear, make it appealing, make it simple, and make it rewarding.

When introducing something new into our lives, especially if it calls for a shift in behavior, we need to follow a process. There are plenty of proven methods out there, but I'm offering you straightforward and practical approaches that have proven more effective in my daily routine. Give them a shot, or feel free to stick to a process that resonates best with you.

a. Repetition Rhythm:

Make it a ritual—repeat the steps for achieving your goal daily for 48 days. Heck, you can even run through it 6 to 9 times each day if that suits you better.

b. Visualize the Victory:

Tackle the process once a day and sprinkle in some mental imagery. This not only plants the process in your subconscious but makes it as natural as your morning coffee routine.

c. Savor the Success:
Watch the results unfold and soak in the satisfaction. It's about relishing the joy in your journey. This subtle shift in mindset will gradually nudge your mental observations into the comfort zone, making it second nature. Get ready to groove into your new habits!

.

Correcting the Old Habits

To effectively amend ingrained habits, a prudent approach involves first delineating a well-defined objective and subsequently embarking on the initiation of a novel course of action.

By establishing a clear and precise goal, one lays the foundation for a purposeful and intentional transformation of old habits. This deliberate and thoughtful methodology serves as a catalyst for change, steering individuals toward a more refined and improved version of themselves.

I recommend that my readers embrace these systematic approach to cultivate wholesome habits and attain their health objectives.

III Overview of SPS Healthy Habits

"The secret of health for both mind
and body is to live in the present
moment wisely and earnestly."

— Buddha

A recent study suggests that adopting healthy habits may not only add valuable years to one's lifespan but also act as a shield against serious illnesses like diabetes. After all, the prospect of gaining an extra decade on this earth is much more enticing when you envision it as an opportunity to truly relish and delight in life!

In the quest for a pristine inner physique, embracing healthy habits becomes paramount. Think about it – just as we value the outer cleanliness of our bodies, ensuring a fresh and inviting aura, shouldn't we extend the same courtesy to our inner anatomy and physiology?

As a note, maintaining outer cleanliness not only makes us approachable to friends (no one wants to enter the realm of stink, right?), but it also doubles as a therapeutic regimen for our inner organs. So, let's not underestimate the power of a good polish – it's not just about smelling good, but also about giving our insides a refreshing cleanse.

In the realm of acupuncture, each main organ is akin to a monarch with its own set of external organs, acting as two-way mirrors. Picture them as the frontline warriors from epic old-age films, armed with spears and shields, not only safeguarding the health of the rulers but also reflecting their well-being. Similarly, these external organs in our body serve as vigilant warriors, defending against external

invaders like germs.
Liver opens in our eyes.
Kidneys listen through our ears.
Heart speaks through our tongue.
Lungs feel with the skin and
Our spleen kisses with the lips.
When water cleans them out,
The kings get their royalties, too.

Picture this scenario: No time for a proper bath, so you settle for a few drops of water here and there. Changing clothes? Just spritz a bit of perfume and call it good. Socks need washing? A couple of drops of water will do the trick. It's a life of constant hustle—eating, traveling, enjoying, sleeping, and chasing that paper - money. Everything else? Fast-tracked. Now, let that sink in for years on end. Ever wonder what our outward appearance would be like?

Now, here's the twist: what if I told you this rapid-fire lifestyle is a mirror to what's happening inside our bodies? Intrigued? Welcome to the surprising world of our anatomy and physiology, where shortcuts reign supreme!

Presenting the game-changers in our quest for a healthy lifestyle—the SPS healthy habits. SPS, shorthand for Super-Powerful-Simple, encapsulates a set of habits deeply rooted in cultures worldwide. These practices aren't groundbreaking discoveries; they've been part of our heritage. However, it's time to shine a spotlight on them and unravel the science behind their efficacy.

Each habit outlined in this book is backed by scientific research, although I won't inundate you with the data here. My focus is on emphasizing the significance of these habits and guiding you through the proper methods in this guide. Consider me your explorer in this wellness journey—I've delved into various customs, comprehended their significance, put them to the test, and now, I'm here to share the wisdom. Let's unlock the secrets to a healthier life together!

Who are the audiences?

These habits are so straightforward that even a toddler could grasp them. No age limits here – after all, isn't age just a number? Absolutely, especially when it comes to health. **Consider these habits as the organic goodness for your well-being. They're like the healthiest snacks for your body, meant for everyone to savor and relish the benefits.** While these practices are for everyone, I specifically want to spotlight:

- The little ones diving into the world of learning. It's the perfect time to instill these habits;
- Parents and grown-ups. Once you experience the perks, you'll become a living example for your kids and others;
- Anyone embracing minimalism, recognizing the power of achieving more with less effort and resources. If you're after the maximum health benefits with minimal fuss, these habits are your golden ticket.

Highlights of this program

- Just six practices that safeguard the essence of our health and stand as vigilant protectors of our internal systems.

- Once adopted, they become lifelong companions, steadfast in their commitment.

- These habits are accessible to anyone, regardless of age, making them suitable for all to embrace and incorporate into their routine.

Essentials

*Sporting a radiant SMILE.** Keep that smile shining bright!.

"Light up a smile on your face to light up happiness among many." ☺

Be mindful to your actions. Be fully present in the moment. Often, we're physically present, yet our minds wander off into the realm of dreams.

"When we start watching what we do, it helps our thoughts to be in the present."

Being yourself. Channel your inner child. Our desires and preferences are deeply linked to our body and mind, so stay open to listening to them.

"Keep your unrestricted mode 'ON' at all times."

Let me share a story about my friend on the train, a bit north of fifty. Her granddaughter urged her to dance, something she'd never attempted. Joining in a few times, she found joy in a simple hip movement. That sparked her interest, leading her to join a dance class for more steps. If it brings you joy, go for it.

Follow your heart and appreciate your delight.

IV Habit 1: Mouth Wash

"Your body is a reflection of your lifestyle."
— **Jack LaLanne**

Gone is the era of early risers and tranquil mornings—today, we're juggling three shifts, drowning in a sea of gadgets, and barely keeping our heads above the flood of information. But, no need to fret.

Enter the game-changer: our mouth-wash technique. Master this routine, and watch as your body realigns itself, finding balance in the dance of Vata, Pita, and Kapha—those dynamic trios of Ayurvedic principles. It's the secret sauce for reclaiming equilibrium, no matter how hectic your schedule may be!

Let's be crystal clear—nothing beats the heavenly embrace of an early, restful night's sleep for your body and mind. It's the best gift you give to yourself. Now, here's the golden nugget: consider this mouthwash method as the perfect complement to turbo-charge your energy levels. It's not a substitute for the bliss of a good night's sleep, but think of it as your trusty sidekick in the quest to revitalize your body and mind.

Right from their initial ventures into face washing and brushing, children should be coached to adopt this technique. They naturally pick up on these habits by watching and emulating the grown-ups around them. Therefore, it falls on the parents to lead by example and personally guide their kids through these routines.

Direction:

- Do mouth was as soon as you wake up and toileting.
- Use this method whenever you do mouthwash.

- During mouthwash, express gratitude to the five elements - Space, Fire, Earth, Air, and Water - for their care. It may sound technical, but appreciate their role in internal and external cleansing.

Technique:

Step 1. Rinsing the mouth

> **Pour water** in your mouth; Lift your face little upwards.

> **Let water flow stiffly** up and down. The water should touch left upper limit of the gums and then right side.

> **Do this way few times** (21 times are good recommendation).

> **Gently blow out the air** from your throat three times (keeping the water in the mouth).

> **Bend down and open your mouth** to throw the water down; note that the mucus from throat may come out. **Open wide** for few more seconds for the saliva flow down.

Note: Initially, you may feel vomiting sensation. By practice, you will get flow and know the method to do it swiftly.

Step 2. Washing the face

> **Take some water on your left hand** and wash your left side of the face from top to bottom.

> ➤ **Take some water on your right hand** and gently wash your right side of the face.

> ➤ **Take some water on your left hand again** and wash the middle face from forehead down till the throat.

Now, wash your face in your normal way and complete.

Dos:

- ✓ Do it with mindfulness.
- ✓ Bring a big smile to your face after face wash.
- ✓ Enjoy the process.
- ✓ Use warm water at body temperature.

Don'ts:

- ☐ Don't use either hot or chill water.

Variations:

- You can perform step 1 and step 2 as separate activities.
- Based on your time schedule, do it individually or together.

Benefits:

- ❖ This habit balances the tridosha (of ayurveda principle) vata, pitta and kapha.
- ❖ While doing it in the early morning, it activates chandra naadi(left side breath) and surya naadi(right side breath) and balances them.
- ❖ This process improves vision and all eye related issues.
- ❖ It improves skin health.
- ❖ This process also helps in immunity through nabhi set. Nabhi is the center of our body; our left and right sides of our body is balanced at nabhi. When

nabhi is at balance, our body's immunity power is high and protects the body from external and internal invasion.

V Habit 2: Squat Toileting

"I don't count my sit-ups. I only start
counting when it hurts because they're
the only ones that count."
— **Muhammad Ali**

It is said that empty your cup before taking any new ideas. This is the most important aspect in any new learning session. This concept is not only applicable for our brain, it is much applicable for our stomach, too.

Understanding the intricacies of the human digestive system provides profound insight into the remarkable journey our sustenance undergoes before being ultimately expelled as waste. Commencing with the ingestion of food through the oral cavity, this intricate process, aptly known as digestion, embarks on a journey that commences at the mouth.

Upon entry into the mouth, essential enzymes intermingle with the masticated food, aided by saliva excreted by the salivary glands. The amalgamation of enzymes and saliva initiates the breakdown of ingested substances, setting the stage for subsequent stages of digestion. Post this oral phase, the transformed alimentary bolus embarks on its automatic traverse down the esophagus, a muscular conduit orchestrating the seamless conveyance of nourishment to the stomach.

Within the stomach's confines, the culinary concoction encounters a medley of imperative enzymes, further refining its composition. This harmonious collaboration between enzymes and stomach facilitates the preparation of the ingested material for its imminent encounter with the small intestine. Upon this culinary transformation, the nutrient-laden mixture is meticulously released at the commencement of the small intestine.

The small intestine, an extraordinary conduit of approximately 5 meters in length, assumes the mantle of extracting vital nutrients from the now-refined concoction. This winding passage orchestrates the absorption of essential elements, setting the stage for the subsequent assimilation of these nutrients into the bloodstream.

Transitioning seamlessly from the small intestine, the residual substance enters the large intestine, a comparably shorter segment measuring around 1.5 meters. Despite its brevity, the large intestine plays a pivotal role in water absorption and the formation of fecal matter, preparing the remnants for their impending exit from the body.

In envisioning this gastrointestinal odyssey as a tube facilitating the transfer of sustenance, the imperative aspect lies in the unobstructed flow of food. Any impediment, whether in the form of waste accumulation or sedimentation, disrupts this delicate equilibrium, hindering the smooth progression of nutrients from the stomach to their ultimate egress.

The digestive process, akin to an intricately choreographed ballet, necessitates an unobstructed path to ensure the unhindered passage of nourishment through its various stages, ensuring the seamless orchestration of this physiological symphony.

The functions of the small and large intestines extend beyond the mere transportation of food; they play a crucial role in the intricate processes of nutrient absorption and waste elimination within our digestive system. The small intestine serves as a vital site for segregating various nutrients from the ingested food chime. This intricate task is facilitated by the presence of villi, small hair-like protrusions lining the intestinal wall, which diligently absorb these essential nutrients. Once absorbed, these nutrients seamlessly integrate into the bloodstream, facilitating their distribution throughout the entire body.

Conversely, the large intestine serves as a key player in the absorption of water and essential vitamins, concurrently filtering water from the chime. The assimilated products, along with water, are then directed to the kidneys for further processing. Subsequently, the solid waste travels through the intestines to reach the rectum. In the rectum, solid waste is collected and subsequently expelled through the anus, completing the intricate journey of food from the mouth to the anus.

The importance of maintaining the cleanliness of this digestive pathway cannot be overstated. The malodorous nature of waste in the toilet underscores the significance of proper intestinal care. Ensuring a smooth flow of digestion and absorption is contingent upon various factors, including dietary choices, exercise routines conducive to digestion, mental well-being, and adequate water intake. Incorporating Ayurvedic principles, such as the consideration of the body's tridosha, further adds depth to our understanding of digestive health.

Central to these considerations is the pivotal role of timely waste elimination, particularly in the early morning hours. Optimal digestive function is not only contingent upon external factors but is significantly influenced by our deliberate attention and commitment to maintaining a healthy elimination routine. Therefore, it is imperative to prioritize this aspect of well-being, recognizing its paramount importance in fostering overall digestive health and, consequently, the broader spectrum of our bodily functions.

As per acupuncture body organ clock, 5am to 7am in the morning belongs to large intestine. If the large intestine is cleaned during this time, it helps to strengthen our guts and to prepare for its run the whole day work.

Our ancestors used a particular method to flush out so that the rectum and anus are naturally strengthened and this process helped to activate all internal digestive system. It's like a triggering internal systems. It's known as SQUAT sitting for toileting.

Ah, a profound exhalation resonates audibly, echoing a sentiment of acceptance. While our generation may not indulge in the luxury of certain practices, let us strive to enhance the well-being of subsequent generations by ensuring they revel in the myriad health benefits.

The squat position, a venerable facet of workouts, stands as an exemplary lower-body exercise, diligently engaging the quadriceps, hamstrings, glutes, and calves. Beyond its prowess in physical conditioning, it exerts a subtle influence on various physiological functions.

In the rustic landscapes of Asia, the tradition of squat-toileting persists steadfastly across all age groups. A stark contrast emerges in urban landscapes, where the advent of chair-sitting toilets, often referred to as western toilets, has relegated the age-old squatting custom to obscurity.

A vivid recollection surfaces of a familial episode at my aunt's abode a decade hence. In the pursuit of constructing a new house, my aunt ardently advocated for the incorporation of a squat toilet in the communal lavatory. A familial divide ensued, with others advocating for the convenience of chair-sitting, or western-style toilets. The impasse escalated to such an extent that my aunt, disheartened by the compromise, abstained from nourishment for two days. Eventually, a consensus was reached – a compromise that yielded a solitary squat toilet outdoors, while the remainder embraced the modern ease of chair-sitting conveniences.

In the annals of history, squat toilets were once commonplace, seamlessly woven into the fabric of daily life. However, their prevalence has waned in contemporary times, supplanted by the ubiquity of western-style conveniences. The evolution of convenience has led to the emergence of two-in-one toilet designs, seamlessly accommodating both sitting and squatting preferences, epitomizing the fusion of tradition and modernity.

Since the time of civilisation, the history gives many examples for squat toilet usages. Toilets with a sitting design have a long history, dating back to as early as 2500 BC in the remains of the Harappan civilization in India. Archaeological excavations provide evidence of the presence of sitting-type toilets in Egypt, also, around 2100 BC. It took many forms and transformations.

In the 19th century, a plethora of advanced methods emerged, contributing significantly to the evolution of the current Western lifestyle. This period witnessed the establishment of one of the most exemplary hygienic practices, although not without its drawbacks. Chief among the concerns was its potential impact on health.

Fast forward to the present day, where a cutting-edge two-in-one method has seamlessly addressed this health-related drawback. This innovative approach incorporates the best elements of the historical practices while mitigating potential health concerns, resulting in a refined and comprehensive hygienic solution.

Therapy Systems:

As per Varma or Marma system, squat sitting induces the

following points:

* Nabhi marma which induces small intestines and large intestines
* Indravasti marma which induces digestive system

As per Acupuncture, squat sitting induces the following points:

According to Ayurveda and LMNT Neurotherapy, assuming a squatting position has the unique ability to harmonize the Chandra Nadi (lunar energy channel) and Surya Nadi (solar energy channel). This traditional wisdom suggests that by adopting this particular sitting posture, an individual can achieve a balance between the subtle energies associated with the moon and the sun.

In the realm of Ayurveda, Chandra Nadi and Surya Nadi are considered integral components of the pranic system, representing the lunar and solar energies, respectively. The practice of squatting is believed to facilitate the alignment and equilibrium of these energies, contributing to an overall sense of well-being and vitality.

In the context of LMNT Neurotherapy, the emphasis is placed on the neurological benefits of squat sitting. This approach views the nervous system as intricately connected to the balance of energies in the body. By adopting the squatting position, it is posited that one can positively influence the neurophysiological pathways associated with Chandra Nadi and Surya Nadi, fostering a state of neurological harmony.

In essence, squat sitting is not merely a physical act; it is a deliberate and intentional practice aimed at attaining a serene balance between opposing forces, as symbolized by the lunar and solar energies. Through this elegantly simple posture, individuals may seek to align themselves with the inherent rhythms of nature, promoting a sense of equilibrium that extends beyond the physical realm into the realms of energy and consciousness.

Technique:

> Gracefully assume a seated position with your legs comfortably folded as you embark on the contemplative act of using the toilet.

> Inhale deeply, allowing the calming breaths to permeate your being, fostering a sense of relaxation. Deliberately observe the gentle ebb and flow of your breath, appreciating the tranquil rhythm.

> Following the squatting posture, gracefully rise from your seat, and engage in the deliberate and controlled movement of opening and closing your anus, repeating this refined exercise three to six times. This mindful practice contributes to a harmonious and mindful approach to bodily functions, promoting a sense of well-being.

Variations:

- Experiment with squatting on two-in-one Western-style toilets for added health benefits
- If squat toilets aren't available, incorporate squat sitting poses into your daily routine, especially before and after using the toilet.

Benefits:

- While squatting, the puborectalis muscle relaxes and rectum straightens. This helps the gravity to pull.
- Easy pose to let the way for the trash to be pulled out by the gravity from rectum to anus.
- It helps to clear all the gases in the abdominal part.
- The pose helps to stretch all the muscles and the

joints of lower part of the body.

❖ Squat position helps thighs to put a gentle pressure on abdomen which takes less time to empty the bowel.

❖ It needs less effort to empty the bowel.

❖ This pose gives a complete body stretch which is good to keep all the internal organs healthy.

VI EXERCISE 3: Method Of Drinking Water

"Sip by sip, you sculpt the river of health that flows through the vessel of your body."

— Ayurvedic Saying

How many of us know that there are methods to drink water? And, how many of us know that the method of drinking water helps us to maintain our healthiness? It is surprising, isn't?

Vedic texts says "**Hail to you, divine, unfathomable, all purifying Waters...**"(Rig Veda).

Seventy percent of our body is made up of water. Our blood also has 70:30 ratio of water. Our body indicates the Earth element out of five elements system. Mother Earth does have 70 percent of water so we! The Water makes the Earth fertile, nutrients, and healthy.

Therapy System:

Five Elements theory

Wood, Fire, Earth, Air and Water are the five elements of five-elements theory. Earth and Water comes as grand-parent and grand-child relationship. Grand-parent controls grand-child.

The Earth controls the Water. However, the Water controls the Fire and the Fire in turn

1. Creates the Earth.

2. Controls the Air and the Air creates the Water.

Knowing our major portion of our body is maintained by water, we should understand its importance in our body. If there is a right maintenance of water in our body, the other elements are to be well-balanced.

There is an age-old saying, "Eat water and drink food" - Sip on your eats and savor your sips.

Prerequisites:

- Let the Water be luke-warm or in body temperature.
- Sitting position is good to consume water.
- Look at the Water and consume.

Technique:

Let's explore the proper way to drink water.

➢ Take the Water in a glass or in a bottle in your left hand.

➢ Sit relax.(Sitting and drinking helps health)

➢ Lift your chin / head little up and open your mouth.

➢ Pour handful of water into the mouth.

➢ Wet your lips slightly with the Water.

➢ Mix saliva into water.

➢ Divide the water into three part and

➢ Gulp three times

This way, most of the water is absorbed by the system in the esophagus itself.

Dos

✓ Keep your body erect, keep the muscles and joints loose and relax.

✓ Look at the Water.

✓ Thank Water for its goodness to our health.

✓ Give a gap of minimum 15 minutes before and after food.

✓ Drinking water in the empty stomach after wake up is good to clean our systems.

✓ When thirsty consume water soon.

Don'ts

☐　Do not drink water when you are angry.

Variations:

- Instead of three gulps, it can be taken up to seven gulps.
- The left leg can be kept little forward than right leg,

Benefits:

- Water balances the other four elements.
- Helps to overcome dehydration.
- Helps to keep the skin shiny.
- All organs energy is balanced.
- This also supports the improvement of the presence of the mind.
- It improves brain functionality.

- It enhances the circulation of blood to various parts of the body.
- It supports our brain cells and improves concentration.
- Balances body and mind

VII Habit 4: Method of Eating Food

"The path to health is paved with choices, and each morsel is a step towards vitality or ailment. Choose wisely."
— Indian philosophy

As we have seen earlier, our digestive system starts from our mouth. Lips, teeth, mouth, salivary glands and saliva, esophagus, mucus, stomach bag, pancreas, spleen, liver, gall bladder, small intestine, large intestine, rectum and anus.

The important function of digestive system is to digest the food that we eat, that is to break into small absorbable parts and absorb the nutrients from the digested food. Later, put away the remains through anus.

How many of us thought that the food what we eat undergoes so many changes to get all the nutrients? The digestive system is the foundational system based on which all other systems, organs and tissues do their work. So, if there is any issue in our body, first system that we need to look into is our digestive system. Though it is a vicious cycle between digestive system and other organs functions, important one be the digestive system.

When we eat food we need not understand all the functions of our digestive system. But, certainly we have to be devoted to give our complete support to the digestive system to complete its obligation successfully.

Look at that crow
Next to it, is a sparrow
There comes a parrot
It brings a walnut
Ready to share shy fully
All eat happily

Look at that cow
Next to it is a goat
There comes a donkey
It brings a bow of grass
Ready to share shy fully
All eat happily

Look at that fly
Next to it is a sweet
There comes an ant
It brings an army
Ready to share shy fully
All eat happily

Ever pondered the idea that our energy could find equilibrium even with a day of no eating? A friend once quipped, "What's the takeaway from life? Let's relish every culinary delight while we're still here."

Some believe life revolves around food, unable to skip a single meal. They're accustomed to indulging in hearty, diverse meals. Heading out for just two hours? They'll seize any chance to chow down, making pit stops at every tempting food stall they spot.

At parties, there's always that group who indulges a bit

extra in the culinary delights. Their taste buds reign supreme, guiding them to savor every flavor, sometimes overriding the sensible signals from their stomachs and digestive systems. It's a delicious struggle between willpower and the irresistible allure of taste!

These situations are taking a toll on their well-being, leading to the emergence of a sizable belly that obstructs their view of their own feet. If we can't grasp the capabilities of our own system, then who can?
Food acts as the spark plug for all our other systems. When there's an excess, it throws off the balance, causing the rest to struggle in carrying out their functions effectively.

In the grand design of our bodies, the brain takes the lion's share of energy, followed by the digestive system. The clever architect of our being arranged it so that when digestion demands energy, other systems graciously hit the pause button and share their resources.

Now, picture this: You decide to go all out on a feast, loading up your stomach. What happens next? Well, all the other systems have to twiddle their thumbs, waiting for digestion to wrap up. But, guess what? Before they can catch a breath, another wave of food crashes in. It's like a chaotic relay race!

In this jumbled scenario, either the other systems reluctantly shift into slow motion, or the digestive system throws in the towel, saying, "Enough of this waiting game, let me take a breather." The result? Digestion goes haywire, absorption becomes a hit-or-miss, and the rest of the systems are left hungry for their much-needed energy fix.

It's a wild ride in the belly carnival!

In the healing wisdom, there's a saying that keeping the stomach 80% full is the key to staying healthy. The concept mirrors what's highlighted in the book IKIGAI, revealing that Japanese centenarians thrive by adopting this practice along with engaging in reasonable and fulfilling daily activities. In the U.S., a similar ethos was discovered through the experiences.

Why settle for less when we're living in the era of abundance? We're all about going big and bold, so why shortchange our stomachs?

Our energy boosters come from the power sources below:
1. Cosmic energy
2. Sun energy
3. Prana energy from air
4. Water energy
5. Food energy

All five elements generously pitch in for our well-being.

When our food portions are on the modest side, it frees up space for other energies to flow through, maintaining that crucial balance in our bodies.

So, cultivating top-notch eating habits isn't just about staying healthy; it's about giving our bodies and minds the royal treatment they deserve in true human style.

Prerequisites:

- Relax for a few seconds
- Keep your thoughts on the food

Technique:

➢ **Serve the food** on the plate.
➢ Look at it and **say thanks to it**.
➢ **Say thanks to the farmer** who produced it and **all others** who helped to bring it **unto you**.
➢ Take a small portion and put into your mouth.
➢ Chew minimum 9 times and mix saliva into it.
➢ Swallow relax and **feel it** reaching **your stomach**.
➢ Continue for the rest of the food.
➢ Once your stomach is full of 80% or capacity of your digestive system, gas would come out as an indicator(Burping).
➢ Be aware that it is the limit of your stomach and stop eating.
➢ It may take 3-4 hours to feel hungry next.

Dos

✓ Eat only when you feel hungry.
✓ Learn to differentiate real hunger and false hunger. During false hunger, drink water to overcome hunger feel.
✓ Feel the rejuvenation of your energy body while eating.
✓ Three meals a day is good.
✓ You shall include your snacks along with healthy portion of your meal.
✓ Colorful plate with different veggies are good.

Don'ts

☐ Don't over feed your stomach.
☐ Don't divert your attention from food using gadgets or gossips while eating.

Benefits:

❖ Improves digestion, energy levels and concentration.

- ❖ Many digestion related disorders will be corrected.
- ❖ Works well to recover diabetes and obese.
- ❖ Balances the energy flow of the body.

VIII Habit 5: Method of Urination

"...What does not belong to health he casts away to a special place, and sends the good wherever it is needed. That is the Creator's decree..."
— **Philippus Aureolus Paracelsus**

Can you imagine anyone genuinely praising the wonderful aroma of urine? Quite a bizarre thought, isn't it?

Now, how about this: Ever heard of a branch of alternative medicine that actually involves using urine as a treatment? It's called Urine Therapy, or uropathy, or even Shivambu.

Believe it or not, this ancient therapeutic method has its origins in Vedic texts. Curious, right?

A research done by Ashok D.B Vaidya in his article called Urine therapy in Ayurveda sites as below:

There are references in the classical texts of Ayurveda on urines from eight animals, including from humans. Their properties and activities are different based on the source. A very interesting reference to human urine as a treatment of cancer is described in a manuscript – Bhrigu Samhita.

The shlokas run like this: "After going to the urinal, one should collect one's midstream urine in a clean vessel. One should take 1 to 2 tola of urine on a fasting stomach for the duration of one mandal (circa 42 days). The regimen of pathya diet and healthy life style has to be followed".

There is also a chapter on auto-urine therapy in an ancient manuscript of Yoga –Damar Tantra, published by Athavale in an Ayurvedic journal (1960). The instructions are similar to those given by Bhrigu. However, the verses numbered 22 and 23 are relevant in view of a case described (vide infra). Therein it is stated that if auto-urine is taken for six months

continuously with Amruta *(Tinospora cordifolia nee glabra)*
mixed in urine, it will make the person free of serious diseases
and s/he will be healthy and happy.
There is also a documented centuries-long and current usage of
auto-urine drinking in Buddhist and Yogic traditions. This is
said to improve resistance to diseases and a sense of well-being.
Hey,cool! I'm not here to sell you on the wonders of urine
therapy, but let's talk about the importance of pee in our
health game.
Think of urine as another form of water – call it **Holy
Water**, if you will.
Just like you chug down water, letting it out is equally
crucial. It's not just about letting it flow; it's about showing
some respect to this *liquid gold.*
Now, adopting a few smart habits for your bathroom
breaks can keep you in the pink of health. Nail these
routines, and you might not find yourself reaching for that
Holy Urine remedy anytime soon. What do you think?

Technique:

> ➤ Move to the toilet as soon as you get a call from
> your bladder.
> ➤ Keep yourself relax.
> ➤ Observe the flow of urine. Color and smell too if
> possible.
> ➤ Allow the bladder to empty completely.
> ➤ Say thanks to the bladder with a broad smile.
> ➤ Open and close your anus and the urine outlet
> point. Contract and loosen the muscles.
> ➤ After urination, drink little water or as needed.

Dos

> ✓ Observe your urine.
> ✓ Be grateful to your excretion system.

✓ Observe the breath that flows to the bottom of your stomach.

✓ Ensure a complete bladder release.

✓ Resist the temptation to rush through the process impatiently.

Don'ts

☐ Avoid the urge to hold until bursting emergency.

☐ Avoid pushing the pee out impatiently

☐ Not to show unhappy face to the smell of your own urine.

Benefits:

❖ The right urination helps to balance the five elements of our body and in turn all the organs.

❖ Relaxes our body.

❖ It helps in overcoming hormonal imbalances and regenerative system disorders.

❖ This method increases the life of kidneys.

❖ This method helps kidney to purify blood properly.

❖ It maintains and keeps our body hydrated.

IX Habit 6: Method of Relaxation

"A healthy outside starts from the inside."

—Ayurveda

My book - *Free Medicine: 6 Super Powerful Simple Health Yoga*, says *"We should spend at least five minutes daily calmly and quietly. This helps to regain our energy levels; it helps to balance our systems, and it also supports our body's ability to heal. This is all about meditation"*.

The book adds, *"The high frequency of beta brainwaves ranges from 12 Hz to 40 Hz. The more we work while being influenced by these waves, the more anxiety, stress arousal, difficulty relaxing, etc., are supposed to affect us. The frequency range of alpha brainwaves is 8 to 12 Hz, which is considered to be moderate. If these brainwaves influence us more, we enter relaxed and passive attention"*.

It also gives a meditation technique along with a simple balancing exercise. You can refer the book, "**FREE MEDICINE: 6 Super Powerful Simple Healthy Yoga Techniques.**"

Our beautiful planet Earth has this awesome natural vibe at 7.8Hz, also known as Schuman's resonance frequency. Now, get this: our brain's frontal lobe is totally on the same wavelength, literally rocking at 7.8Hz, syncing up with Mother Earth. When we're grooving to this frequency, it's like a VIP pass to the ultimate healthy mind and body state. But here's the deal – the moment we lose that connection with Mother Earth, our health takes a bit of a nosedive.

So, if you're all about staying healthy and rolling in the good vibes (and who isn't?), you've gotta vibe with Mother

Earth. The secret sauce? Relaxation is key, and if you're feeling extra fancy, throw in some meditation for that ultimate mind-body sync. It's not just about health; it's about wealth – the kind that starts with a happy, resonating you!

Relaxation holds the same level of importance as proper nutrition and regular exercise for both our bodies and minds. Allow me to share the daily hustle of one of my Indian associates who practices therapeutic methods, unveiling a lifestyle that many of us can relate to.

At the crack of dawn, her day kicks off at 4:30 am, navigating through kitchen chores until 5:30 am, seamlessly transitioning into the role of getting her kids ready for school by 6:30 am. By 7:30 am, she's diving into the dual tasks of preparing breakfast and lunch for herself and her partner, all while overseeing household support to maintain a spick-and-span living space.

The dash to the office begins by 8:30 am, slightly tardy at times due to the morning juggle, but the real pressure intensifies upon reaching her workplace by 9:30 am. The workday, extending until 6 pm, offers scarce moments for personal breaks, with quick dashes for lunch and nature's calls.

She candidly admits to experiencing genuine work pressure, juxtaposed with colleagues who feign busyness, a perilous charade more insidious than the real work-related stress.

Homecoming at 7 pm marks the start of the evening routine – refreshing conversations with the family until 8:30 pm, followed by dinner. Post-dinner, the meticulous cleanup and preparation for the upcoming day persist until 10 pm, culminating in a well-deserved descent into slumber.

Even amidst this chaotic schedule, she manages to carve out a precious 30 to 60 minutes for relaxation, a time she dedicates to family, mobile conversations, and social media updates. However, it's evident that genuine personal relaxation, the kind that replenishes the soul, remains a fleeting luxury.

In the grand scheme of things, taking a moment for oneself becomes a sacred indulgence, a necessity echoing through the demands of the modern human experience.

From the littlest kiddos to the wisest folks around, we're all hooked on something, always plugged into the mobile or web scene. Whether we're laughing at fun videos, hunting down new cooking recipes, or diving into the depths of thesis research, it's a digital world we're living in. Strolling down the street, stepping onto the school or college campus, even out for a morning walk - the mobile is our ever-present companion. Music, videos, self-help goodies – you name it, it's all right there in our pocket. Free time? What's that?

But let's talk about real relaxation. It's not just about giving our bodies a break; our minds need it too. We've got to hit pause on the constant churn of our mental processors each day. It's like a refreshing reset button for our minds, clearing out the clutter and that pesky thought smog that builds up. Let's find that sweet spot between the digital buzz and a mental breather – the key to rejuvenation for mind and body alike.

Direction:

- ❖ Sitting calm.
- ❖ Doing any healthy hobbies.
- ❖ Writing.
- ❖ Drawing / Painting.
- ❖ Walking

- ❖ Smiling
- ❖ Exercises / Yoga

Indulge in the art of relaxation through the exquisite techniques presented above, each a standalone sanctuary or a harmonious fusion of tranquility. Whether you're crafting prose or gracing the world with your radiant smile, these methods are your exclusive pathways to relaxation, whether pursued as pastimes or as a respite from the daily grind.

Embark on a journey of rejuvenation, elegantly woven into your work routine. For every two hours of dedicated effort, treat yourself to the sublime practice of five minutes of relaxation, an oasis in the midst of your bustling endeavors. Embrace this refined approach, where the symphony of work and relaxation creates a masterpiece of balance and well-being.

Technique:

- ➢ **Sit down**, comfortably. Sukasana is good;
- ➢ **Or Sit on the chair**.
- ➢ Keep your gadgets away.
- ➢ Close your eyes and witness your breath for a few seconds.
- ➢ Open your eyes and start your whatever relaxation technique you want to follow.
- ➢ Continue to 5 minutes.
- ➢ Bring a big smile on your face and complete it.
- ➢ Move on to your regular work.

Variations:

- ■ Combine the techniques.
- ■ Visualization - closing the eyes and visualizing

your hobby

Benefits:

- ❖ This habit helps in calming down your mind.
- ❖ It improves memory power.
- ❖ It builds skills to manage your pressure.
- ❖ It extends self-awareness.
- ❖ It helps to focus in the present.
- ❖ This habit increases innovation and creative power.
- ❖ It extends tolerance and strength of physical body as well as mind.

X Programming your time and mind

"As is the macrocosm, so is the microcosm. As is the cosmic body, so is the personal body. As is the atom, so is the universe"
— Upanishads

Engage in activities that fuel both your body and mind with vitality, steering clear of anything that leaves you feeling depleted. These six potent and super simple habits are meticulously designed to cultivate an energetic and vibrant flow, enhancing both your physical and mental well-being.

Discover the art of straightforward techniques, ensuring an effortless and enjoyable practice. I recommend revisiting and mastering these habitual techniques multiple times to truly embrace their benefits. Elevate your energy, embrace wellness, and relish the journey!

In no time, these habits will seamlessly integrate into your daily routine. At the outset, a bit of mindful effort is all it takes. With a worthwhile goal and the determination to reach it, there's always a path to success!. If there is a will, there is a way, isn't it?

Let's Get Some Self-Motivation

Back in my elementary school days, there was this teacher who had a knack for keeping us on our toes. Picture this – it was the '80s, when parental focus on formal education wasn't as intense. In those days, teachers went the extra mile, literally, visiting homes to round up kids and bring them to school.

Now, this particular teacher had a go-to example to explain why we needed to stay engaged in our studies. Curious students, a bit puzzled about the purpose of it all, would often ask, "Why should we bother with all this learning, Teacher?"

In the charming vernacular of that era, it was a time when bell-bottoms were cool, and neon was in. Fast forward to today, and that teacher's response echoes in my mind: "Alright, kiddos, imagine you're on a journey – a journey to discover the incredible world of knowledge. And guess what? Each lesson is like a treasure chest waiting to be unlocked. So, saddle up, because the adventure of a lifetime is happening right here in our classroom!"

My teacher used to drop these wisdom bombs like no other. Picture this: a sparrow, cruising through life, not stressing about food for a hot minute. But here's the kicker – it never sits on its feathery behind doing nothing. Then, there's the ant squad – tiny food ball enthusiasts who clock in 24/7, not just for a snack but to tidy up the Earth. They're basically the neat freaks of the insect world.

And oh, don't get me started on butterflies. Have you ever seen those majestic creatures emerging from a cocoon? Life-changing stuff, I tell you. Imagine if they decided, "Nah, I'm good staying as a caterpillar forever." Total game-changer for Mother Earth, right?

Now, let's talk about the eagles ruling the skies. Will anything get changed, if that eagle on the sky doesn't fly up? Well, will there be any change, if the jungle king doesn't get crowned? Groundbreaking or what? And the jungle kings – they've got their crowns for a reason.

And, she used to complete saying, "So we, human need to improve our wisdom; let's start it with the school".

Here's the real kicker, though. All these creatures live in the present moment. No crystal ball gazing for them. They live their life complete. Fish swim, birds soar, and animals strut – no ant is caught slacking, not even the queen bees. Yet, here we are, the supposedly superior beings, getting tangled in the web of money and status. It's like we signed up for a race without knowing where the finish line is, and now we're too deep to hit the brakes and figure out what's what. Time for a reality check, folks.

Babies instinctively follow their consciousness, finding prosperity in simple joys like smiling, laughing, and taking things in stride. Their cries serve as a natural expression of needs. In winter, they embrace activity, while summer invites rest. Yet, as they grow, the connection with nature and innate creativity often gives way to the trappings of our supposedly advanced culture.

In our modern lifestyle, even basic natural activities essential for well-being are sometimes disregarded. Take sneezing, for instance: scientific explanations abound, yet many block their noses when the urge arises.

While some may perceive it as a matter of decorum, it's crucial for health to embrace sneezing as a natural, body-initiated cleansing process. Broad-mindedness is key, acknowledging both our own and others' sneezes as a fundamental aspect of nature, irrespective of external circumstances.

Embracing these fundamental SPS habits is like donning life-jackets for your well-being—nature's way of ensuring our health. In every culture, similar SPS habits abound, and this book serves as a guide to understanding their significance. My aim is to curate the most impactful habits, creating a path to reconnect with nature.

As we express gratitude to the external world—planting trees, acknowledging the universe, or sharing smiles with neighbors—let's not forget to cultivate gratitude for our internal existence. It all begins with these super powerful yet simple habits we adopt and consistently follow.

If the essence of gratitude hasn't fully resonated with you in the preceding six healthy habits outlined in this book, consider revisiting and immersing yourself in their core message. These habits have the transformative power to reshape your external world—enriching your happiness, success, and relationships. Restart your journey through this book, and let the positive change unfold.

Feel free to enhance these habits or dive into the essence of this guide, centered on the pivotal concept that **achieving balance in the five elements of our body is key**. Cultivate these habits as part of your daily routine, crafting a lifestyle that harmonizes these elements.

Infuse your routine with additional wellness practices to ensure equilibrium in your body's core elements. In the end, **the ultimate goal is to radiate health and well-being**.

Pursuing a routine is very much like sowing seeds. Embarking on a routine is akin to planting seeds for your future. You get to decide what you want to cultivate, planting the seeds with a vivid vision of your desired outcome. No need to stress about the twists and turns; it's about infusing your journey with insight to fulfill your purpose. Just like tending to a garden, pluck out any weeds you come across.

Success entirely depends on what you believe is possible for you. Success hinges on what you believe is within your grasp. Your external experiences merely mirror what's in your mind. If you do not vibe with your current situation, a simple change of perspective can work wonders. Expect the best, express gratitude to your mind and the Universe (or

God), and watch your outer experiences align with your positive mindset.

Recognize that every aspect of your life propels you toward your goals, especially when it comes to the ultimate goal: being healthy. After all, **health is wealth**!

Consider the tenacity of Thomas Edison, who reportedly took 10,000 attempts to create a working light. Most would have thrown in the towel after a fraction of that, but Edison remained fervently committed. Perhaps he knew he had to discover 9,999 ways not to make a light before reaching his goal. **Apply this resilient mindset to elevate your health and fitness journey**.

XI FAQs

"The groundwork for all
happiness is good health."

— Leigh Hunt

<u>What is the best age for these habits to start with?</u>

Embarking on this journey is fantastic from the very start, say, from the age of infant, but the beauty lies in starting whenever the timing clicks. . Whether you're a savvy grown-up passing on your pearls of wisdom or a fresh-faced learner soaking it all in, this exchange becomes a priceless gem intricately woven into the tapestry of life. Every age is ripe for the wisdom dance, creating a symphony that enriches the soul.

<u>Do I need to follow any specific diet?</u>

Indulging in wholesome, natural eats is a great call, but here's the twist – how we approach our meals might just steal the spotlight from what's on the plate. Dr. Robert M. Nerem's rabbit rendezvous spilled the beans: the social vibe during chow time can be a game-changer for our well-being. So, as you dig into your grub, channel your inner zen – aim for a cool, collected, and maybe even blissful state. After all, there's wisdom in the age-old saying: "Sip on your eats and savor your sips."

<u>I have an acute illness. Can I follow this program?</u>

These habits are to create a healthy body and mind. So, yes, you can start to get in to a healthy journey.

<u>How about chronic cases? Can I follow this program?</u>

These habits are to create a healthy body and mind. So, yes, you can start to get in to a healthy journey.

<u>They all seem to be so short and regular. Do they work?</u>

They are simple and sample. Our body needs bending or stretching to keep it active and healthy. Our body's impulse rate is around 100m per second. It means any impulse created in any body part reaches another end within 1/100th second. So if any good feel stretch is done, it just needs a few seconds to convey its blessings.

Are there any recommended stress management techniques as part of a healthy habits?

When your body is in top shape, it lightens the load on your mind. Dive into 'FREE MEDICINE: 6 Super Powerful Simple Health Yoga Techniques' for easy methods to tackle stress head-on!

How can I improve my sleep quality for better overall well-being?

A sound body leads to a healthy mind, making it the optimal path to enhance sleep quality

How do I strike a balance between work, personal life, and self-care in the pursuit of a healthy lifestyle?

Set clear boundaries to prevent burnout. Treat self-care as non-negotiable. Allocate quality family time. And regularly assess and adjust your balance as needed. Goal setting and the process to achieve it helps.

Are there any common pitfalls to avoid when adopting healthy habits?

Overambitious Start, All-or-Nothing Mentality and Lack of Patience are common while adopting healthy habits. Start with sustainable changes; embrace progress and results may take time, stay committed.

How do I navigate social situations and gatherings while maintaining healthy habits?

Here are some tips:

Plan Smart: Eat balanced beforehand to avoid overeating.

Stay Strong: Politely say no to unhealthy choices.

BYO Healthy: Bring a nutritious dish to share.
Body Awareness: Stop eating when full; listen to cues.
Connect, Not Consume: Focus on connections, not just food.

<u>**What are the long-term benefits of consistently practicing healthy habits?**</u>

Consistently practicing healthy habits yields lasting benefits, such as increased energy, improved mood, enhanced immunity, reduced risk of chronic diseases, better sleep, and a prolonged, higher quality of life.

<u>**Do you have more questions or need help customizing this program to your goals and situation?**</u>

Reach out to me at graceprabhamenmai@gmail.com

XII. Summary

"To ensure good health: eat lightly, breathe deeply, live moderately, cultivate cheerfulness, and maintain an interest in life."

— William Londen

In a distant realm, an emperor ruled in opulence, his people basking in happiness and vitality. The monarch had a charismatic yet challenging son, whose life's current diverged from his childhood companions.

Despite the daily grooming of good habits, the prince found himself at odds, expressing his frustration to his father. "Why this relentless discipline everywhere?" he questioned. "I can't seem to adhere to any of it."

The discerning king, rather than reprimanding, silently observed and devised a plan. Seeking the counsel of a wise courtier, he tasked the sage with enlightening his son on the importance of cultivating habits.

Taking the prince on a journey to a lush forest, the wise man pointed to a canal sustaining the greenery. "Could we redirect this water to the other side?" he inquired. The prince agreed, but questioned the purpose, highlighting the uselessness of the weeds on the opposite side.

As they strolled, they encountered a leak in the canal. The prince, recognizing the potential consequences, joined the wise man in fixing it. Seated under a tree, the wise man drew parallels, likening good habits to the canal water. "Correct deviations, or they'll breed weeds instead of benefits," he advised.

Transitioning to the essence of health, the narrative delves into the importance of body movement, mental presence, and embracing a holistic approach. It stresses the reader's agency, urging them to convert understanding into action, starting with a single pivotal habit.

Give your muscles the stretches they crave and your joints the bends they need. Keep your mind firmly rooted in the present – a recipe for health and happiness. With the wisdom I've shared, the experiences I've lived, and the experiments I've undertaken, the keys to your well-being are now in your hands.

It's time to turn understanding into action. Remember, even the smallest step is a major health victory. Identify that one pivotal habit and kick start your journey. These habits seamlessly weave into your daily routine, enhancing your health in countless ways.

Just like eating, bathing, and sleeping, using our body to its full potential is essential for both physical and mental well-being. Opt for personal effort over reliance on external aids – it's a holistic approach that pays off in the long run.

Embrace these Super Powerful Simple habits, and complement them with essential, no-frills exercise techniques outlined in my book, **"<u>Free Medicine: 6 Super Powerful Simple Health Yoga Techniques</u>"**.

These straightforward yet impactful routines are non-negotiable for your body's well-being. Elevate your health game by incorporating these minimalistic exercises into your routine, as detailed in the pages of my book. Your body deserves the best, and it starts with mastering the simplicity of these indispensable practices.

I've just scratched the surface, highlighting some key perks of these habits. However, there's a wealth of profound benefits waiting for you to uncover through your own experience. Consider these six SPS healthy habits as your passport to a drug-free voyage—it's either cost-free medicine or a medicine-free adventure. Get ready to seize control of your well-being and embark on a journey to a healthier, vibrant you!

Vaazhga Valamudan— Long live with all the richness of life.

Acknowledgement

Thanks to the Divine Universe for giving me this fantastic opportunity to be an author.

Developing a concept into a book is not easy. The experience is both challenging and rewarding. A word of appreciation is like a world of strength in a time of need. I got appreciation continuously from family – parents, husband and daughters, friends, and mentors. I am here because of them. I thank you all.

I especially want to thank my friends - well wishers who directly or indirectly impacted my positive progress. All your belief on myself, helped me to reach here who I am today. THANK YOU ALL ONCE AGAIN.

I want to express my gratitude to EVERYONE who has ever encouraged me or taught me something. I heard it all, and it was meaningful to me.

My GRATITUDE and a bunch of thanks to you, my readers, for taking the time out to read
"FREE MEDICINE - 6 SPS Healthy Habits"

for your healthy life. I genuinely believe that you have noteworthy actionable health habits that will emphatically help your everyday life to stay healthy and positive.

Shower your appreciation

May I request one minute more of your time?

If you have enjoyed this book, please consider showing appreciation by rating and reviewing "***FREE MEDICINE - 6 SPS Healthy Habits***" on Amazon.

Reviews, ratings and shares are the golden support to authors. They are a colossal help for growing authors like me, who are due for a billion followers. Your review will encourage many to practice these healthy habits and be happy & healthy.

Love you all,
Grace Prabha

RETURN GIFT!

I have created a special Telegram channel for my readers of this book who have reached so far, as a note of thanks for your time and effort. I invite you to my telegram channel, where I share periodic health tips. Only channel members will get a discussion group to answer all your health queries. I will share therapy tips for acute issues of health and mind. Please join the channel using the following link.

"Online Health Consultation - Alternative Therapy Methods"
You are welcome to get in touch with me.

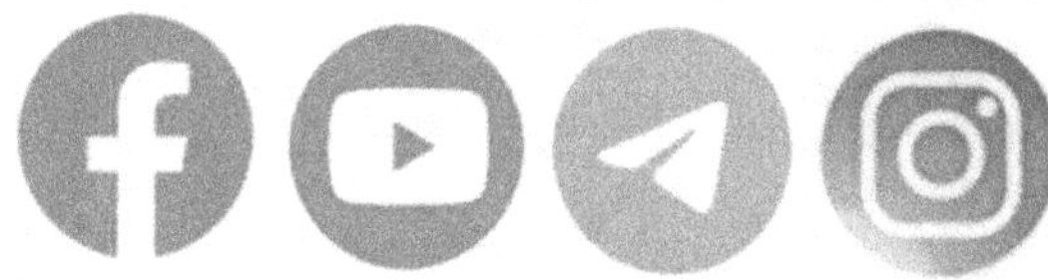

@GracePrabhaMenmai

MY WAY OF HOLISTIC THERAPY

My holistic therapy solutions include

- **LMNT Neurotherapy**
- **Dr. Bach Flower Therapy**
- **Acupuncture**
- **Traditional Energy Medicine**
- **Electro Homeopathy**
- **Reiki Healing**
- **Quantum Healing and**
- **Counseling**

Several benefits of the above therapies and remedies are:

- **Treating acute and chronic issues**
- **Discovering 'Your inner self'**
- **Gaining clarity about 'What you want in life'**
- **Set 'Achievable Goals'**
- **Making 'Empowering Decisions'**
- **Tapping 'Blind Spots and Grow' as a Person**

Over the last few years, alternative therapies have become one of the best ways to create positive changes and lasting results in a healthy life.

You may reach out to me to get the testimonies of these therapies.

If you or someone known to you need therapies or if you want to know more about treatments, do reach out

to me over email at GracePrabhaMenmai@gmail.com.